Malnutrition and Nutrient Deficiency

Knowing more about "Hidden Hunger"

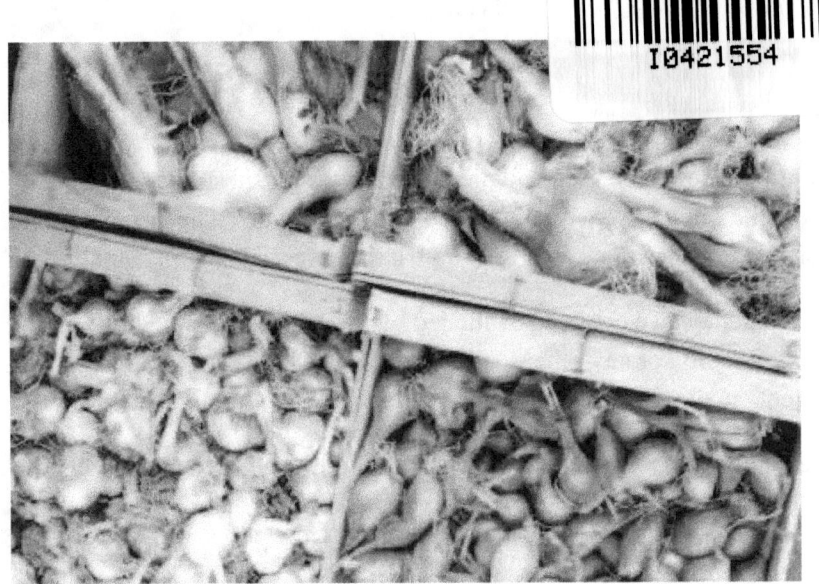

Healthy Learning Series

Dueep Jyot Singh

Mendon Cottage Books

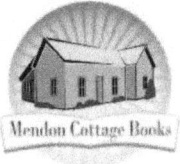

JD-Biz Publishing

Our books are available at

1. Amazon.com

2. Barnes and Noble

3. Itunes

4. Kobo

5. Smashwords

6. Google Play Books

Table of Contents

Introduction

You consider yourself to be a very health conscious person, eating the right foodstuffs, at the right time. However, you have been noticing of late that you get tired easily. You are pale, and feel that subject. You do not feel hungry, very often. You may also suffer from giddiness.

By evening, you're so tired that you have absolutely no patience and inclination to be nice to the rest of the family and you snap at them at the slightest procreation! Naturally the family is at a loss to understand your unusual behavior.

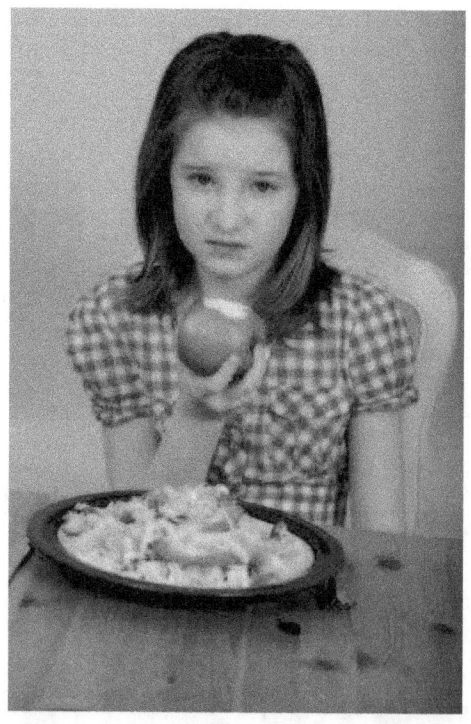

On the other hand, let's take the example of your once happy go lucky teenager. One evening, while playing basketball, she felt dizzy and fell down. Also, her grades which were quite good, in the past have started falling down because according to her she cannot concentrate. Her attention span has shortened considerably. She is very easily distracted, much more than what is normally in a normal teenager!

Both of these examples may be unrelated, but the underlying reason for both of them is the same. You as well as your teenager are suffering from what is normally called "hidden hunger."

This is not an eating disorder, which is self-inflicted, like bulimia or anorexia. This is micronutrient deficiency. This is one of the most important and worrisome of all the public health problems all over the world today. Did you know that 47% of the people, even in well-developed nations are suffering from this micronutrient deficiency?

You may tell yourself, how can that be, you have been eating well and you have been eating often. But what have you been eating? Processed foods? Foods which have been treated in such a manner that all the micronutrients have been removed beforehand, and other supporting additives being placed in those foods instead?

Many of the foods which we eat today are lacking in the essential minerals and vitamins, which are necessary to keep the body functioning properly. These micronutrients include iodine, zinc, iron, and vitamin A.

Hidden Hunger Explained

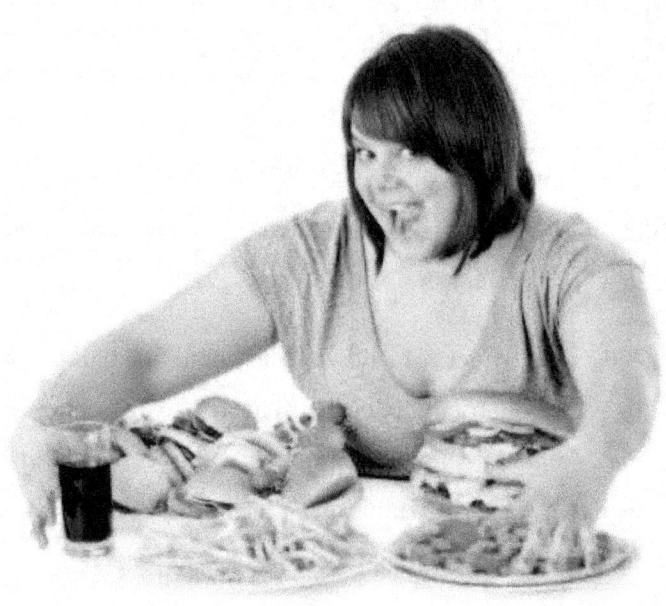

The quantity is astounding, but what about the quality?

Many of us can consider ourselves fortunate, because we have enough of money to eat whatever we want, whenever you want. Most of us usually indulge in overeating as far as food is concerned. We are never hungry and therefore we assume that our food is adequate, even in terms of "quality."

That is because we have loaded up our plates and filled our stomachs with all those foods which we like to eat for breakfast, brunch, lunch, snacks, dinner, and everything else in between. But here we didn't bother much to

---

check about the quality of the food which we have been eating, even though the quantity is eye-catching!

Recent research has shown that *two thousand million* people across the world do not get enough of iron from their food. 1000 million people do not get adequate iodine. Hundred million people have inadequate intake of vitamin A.

Iron, iodine, and vitamin A are the three important nutrients that control the critical functions of development, growth and the performance of all the systems in our body. These nutrients are required in very small amounts, - that is why there are called micronutrients-but they are necessary to keep you healthy and fit.

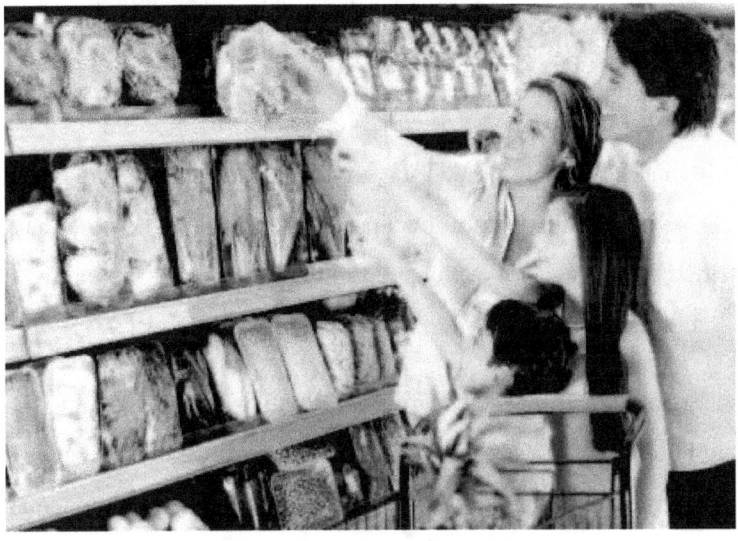

Buying natural and organic foods means that you're less likely to suffer from a micronutrient deficiency.

All these cannot be obtained through supplements, and vitamins, however much the pharmaceutical companies persuade you otherwise. They can only be taken directly through the food, and these natural forms of vitamins are going to be assimilated directly in your system.

I know of a relative who has got into the habit of eating vitamins and supplements, as a substitute for natural meals. She says that is the way in which she is getting all her minerals and vitamins when she doesn't get from her normal meals. Which, as I said before, she skips very often.

So the moment she skips her lunch, breakfast, or dinner she's going to pop three vitamins, four mineral supplements, either in liquid form or in powdered form, and any latest star endorsed product under any brand name, which is been showing ever so often on the TV today.

And she's happy that she is getting her necessary daily quota of vitamins, minerals, proteins, carbohydrates, and essential nutrients.

Don't be like my aunt. Be sensible and remember that normal food, especially that which is natural, homegrown, garden grown, and definitely not processed is the healthiest food available to you. It is going to have all the essential micronutrients which are going to keep your system working properly and in a healthy fashion.

An inadequate intake of all these micronutrients is going to affect all of us – young and old – seriously. When we are young, it is possible that we are not going to see the immediate aftereffects of such a deficiency, immediately. But the cumulative effect is going to go on and on as time goes by, and as we get older.

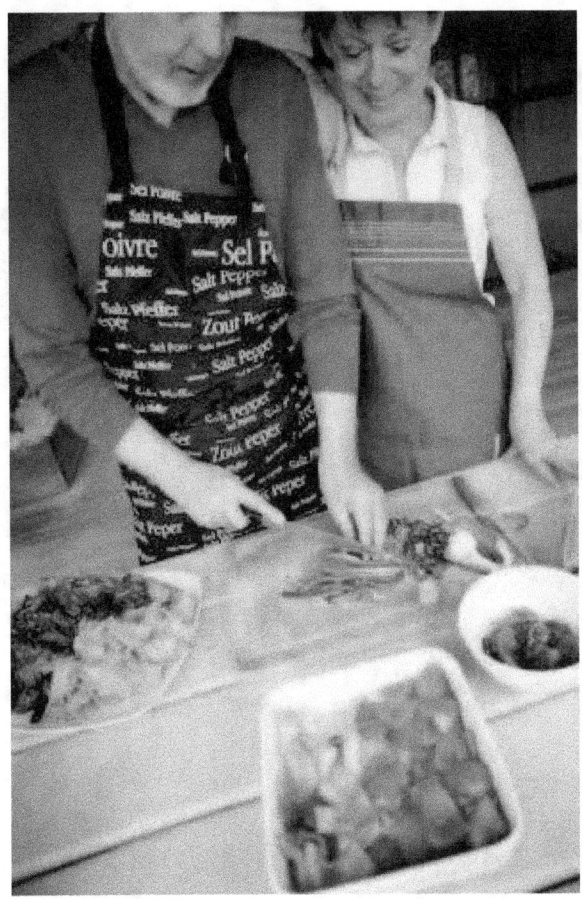

Naturally as we age, we may lose our youthful resilience with the passing of time. Our immunity system is also going to get weaker, especially if we did not have a nutritious diet, when we were young. And above that, if we are suffering from micronutrient deficiency, by the time we reach middle age, we may be suffering from a number of problems, which could so easily have been avoided if we had eaten a sensible diet since childhood.

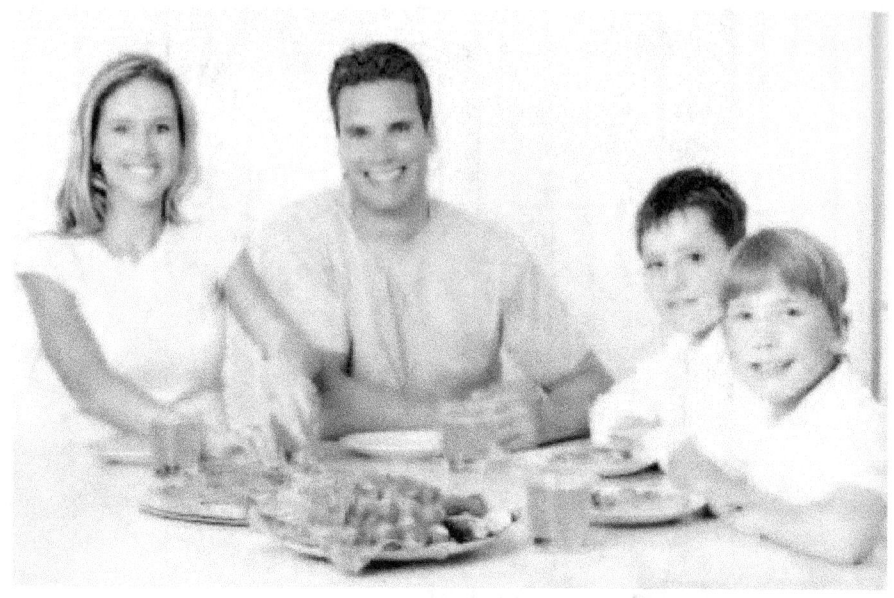

A sensible diet substantially decreases your risk of having a micronutrient deficiency problem.

The term "hidden hunger" has been coined by James Grant of the UNICEF who said that micronutrient deficiency gnaws at the core of health and not below the belly. That is why it is called "hidden hunger".

The Importance of Micronutrients

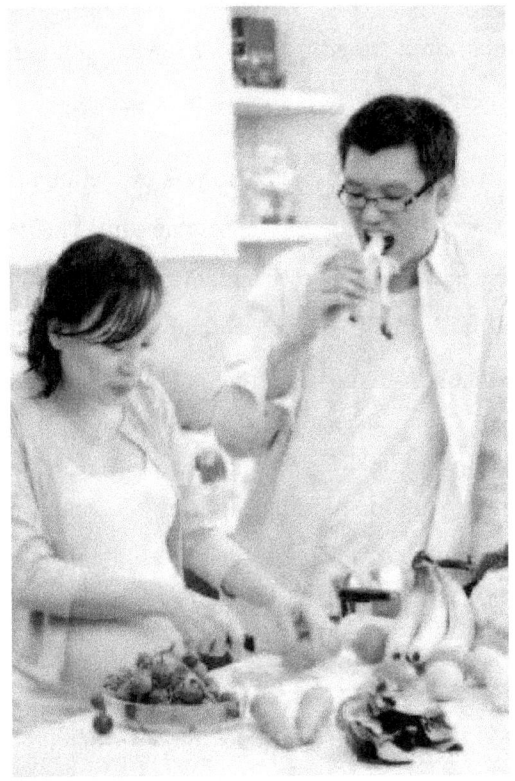

Sensible and health-conscious parents who know about the right things to eat are going to have healthier children.

So your teenager's poor performance at school, and at play could be a result of iron deficiency and vitamin A deficiency. Your lethargy is caused by vitamin and mineral deficiency.

So naturally, you want to know why these minerals and vitamins, even though they are needed in just small quantities are so essential for your good health? Did you know that expectant mothers who did not eat plenty of iron/iodine in their diets will have children, whose brain is not properly developed? Such children are going to have lower intelligence levels. There are also going to perform poorly in their school sessions.

When I told this to one of my friends who was expecting her young one, she told me chirpily that yes, her doctor had told her this. And the doctor had put her onto a very expensive course of Iron tablets. Naturally, she was very indignant when I told her that the iron which her body needed and her baby needed had to be taken from a natural diet, and not from Iron tablets.

What did I know, I didn't have a Medical Degree. Her doctor knew best. I decided to keep shut. And today, little Melinda is seven years old, and her mother is very disappointed due to her lack of academic progress. I just look at Melissa when she starts to complain to me. I don't need to tell her "I told you so."

The necessary food items which she needed to take in abundance was poultry, fish, and red meat. Beans, spinach, and other leafy vegetables, seafood, apricots, raisins, and pork were excellent sources of iron. But she would rather take iron tablets.

But then the world is made up of stubborn fools who are not going to take good advice, based on knowledge and experience, just because it hasn't been backed up by a Medical Degree.

Meat was not an integral part of the diet in the East, in ancient times. At that time they made do with green leafy vegetables, beans, and lentils. As time went by, meat began to get incorporated slowly and steadily in the diet of people in the East, but even then, women did not eat it, because it was supposedly a "strong and hot" food.

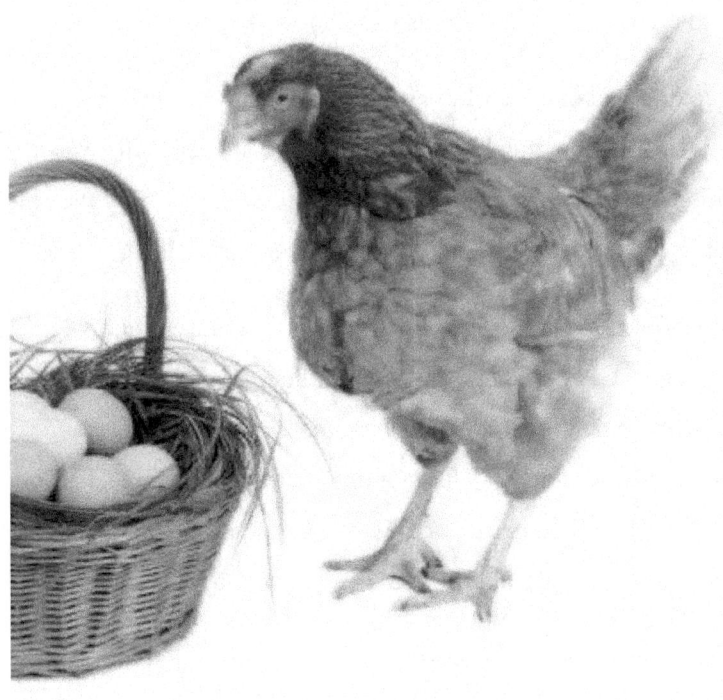

Consider eggs to be an excellent complete food.

This natural prejudice of women not eating meat and eggs is still prevalent in many parts of the world today, especially in countries where ancient traditions prevail even in the 21st century.

However, this rule was relaxed only when a woman was expecting a child. She was then fed meat, chicken, eggs, and other food items on high-protein, so that if she gave birth to a warrior, he would be strong and sturdy!

This reminds me of a really amusing incident, recounted to me by my grandmother. Most of the women of her generation did not eat eggs, meat, and chicken because these meat items were normally kept for the menfolk.

She was recounting about one of the soldiers under my grandfather's command. The British medical officer had told the soldier – this was in the 30s – that his wife was very weak and she needed building up, if the child had to survive. Otherwise she would suffer from a miscarriage.

The soldier spoke in his rustic vernacular – the officers were quite familiar with the language and could curse and yell in the rural and bucolic manner born – "Sir, this woman is a very foolish woman. She does not eat chicken. Her mother did not eat chicken. Her grandmother did not eat chicken. She will not eat meat. If I force her to eat this, she says that she is going to suffer from nausea. She is a very stubborn foolish woman. So what do I do, sir?"

The Medical officer was a very sensible man. He immediately told him to go to the vet and get a syringe, in which medicines were injected in the Regiment's horses!

And then he had to take that huge syringe back home and tell his wife that okay, if she was not going to eat chicken soup, because she felt nauseated, the doctor had given him full permission to inject a syringe full of chicken soup, right into her, three times a day!

The woman immediately added meat to her diet, as quiet as a mouse, when she saw that huge syringe being waved before her eyes.

And she had a very healthy son. Naturally, the other women of the village immediately decided that they did not want to get injected with hypodermic needles full of chicken soup and make sure that they had properly cooked meat regularly when they were expecting babies.

So, a little bit of common sense and a little bit of ancient psychology can do wonders. It also is able to provide all the necessary micronutrients needed to keep expectant mothers healthy, and thus have healthy offspring.

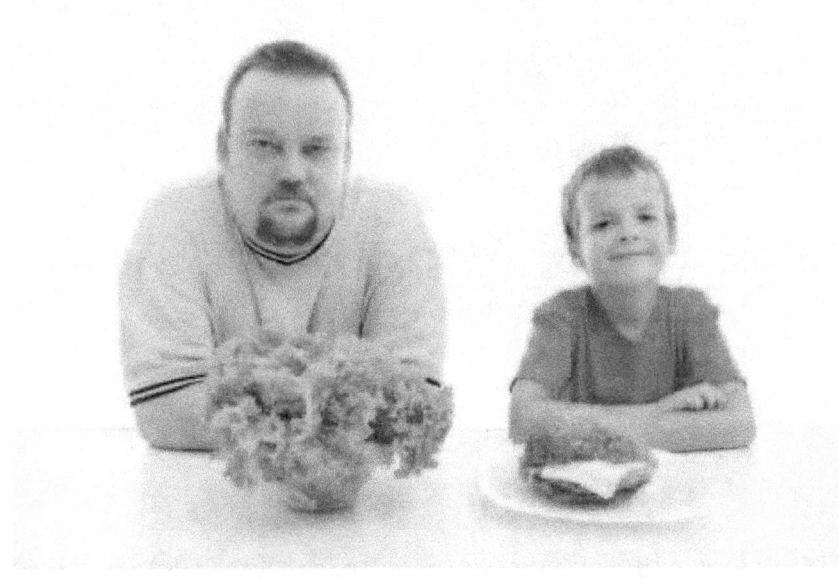

This may be a funny picture, but the kid is going to suffer from a potential micronutrient deficiency in the future. That is because he is not eating the right kinds of micronutrient rich food items.

So if you are complaining that your child is not doing so well academically, or cannot concentrate in his studies, take a good look at yourself. You are to blame. If you had an Iron deficiency during the time you are expecting your child, naturally, he would be born iron deficient. His brain would not have had the opportunity or chance to develop in a healthy and natural manner, poor kid!

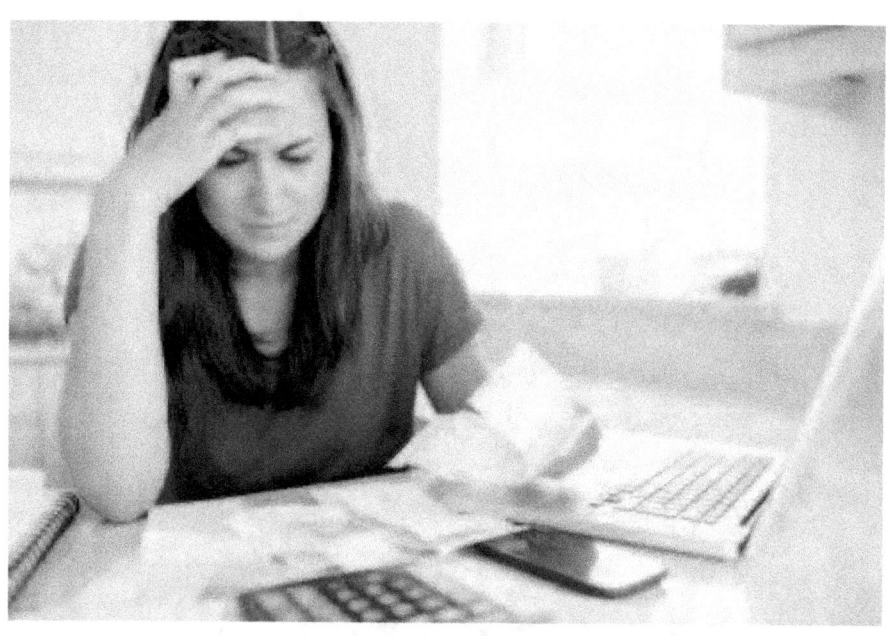

If you find it difficult to concentrate, and are feeling lethargic, it is possible that you are suffering from some sort of deficiency, whether micro or macro.

This little child is also going to have a very low hemoglobin count and he is going to be prone to anemia. This is indicative of iron efficiency. Just 7 g of iron needed for a baby per day could make all the difference between an intelligent child, and in not so intelligent one. A normal dose for a normal human being is 12 g per day, which he needs to eat every day, in his food and not in supplement tablets.

This deficiency naturally would be aggravated, with a poor intake of iron rich foods, after he was born, and in the first few years of childhood. You are going to be surprised to know that children who live next to the sea, and have plenty of seafood and iodine are considered to be more intelligent, healthier and with a stronger immunity system than those children who live in the interior of the country.

Iodine deficiency

Children who suffer from iodine deficiency are technically and medically called Cretins. Unfortunately, this term has become a pejorative term, and an epithet to insult anybody with whom you have had an argument, or whom you want to describe is a total moron.[1]

The children are also going to have muscle disorders as well as speech and hearing defects. They may also suffer from infantile paralysis.

---

[1] This is what I usually did when I was confronted with fools, but being a very brought a person, I never used hateful words like cretin and moron. I just murmured "iodine deficient Homo sapiens" into my files, and was satisfied that not many understood that one of the inefficient deadwoods in the organized patient had just been described comprehensively and thoroughly.

Vitamin A Deficiency

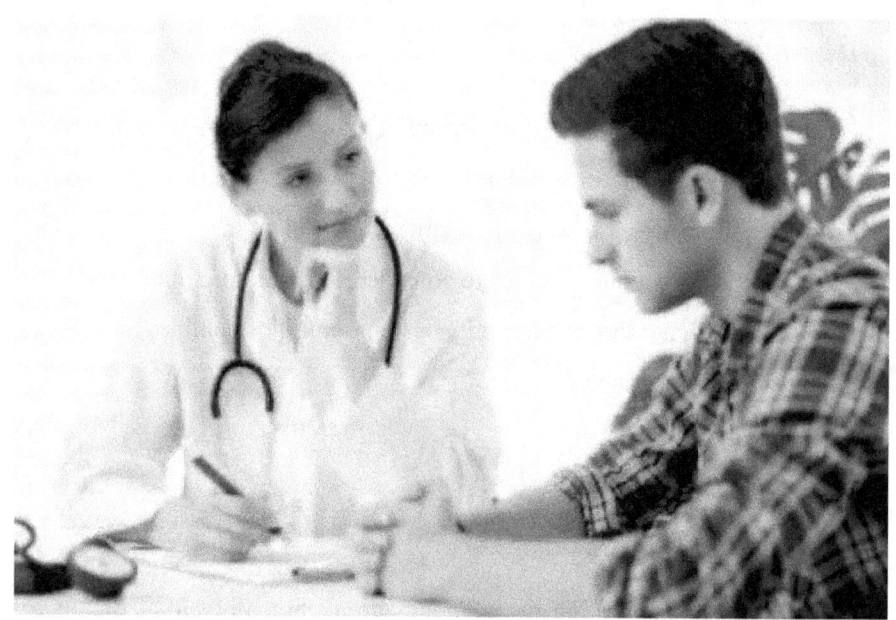

Your eye problems can be partially attributed to a vitamin A deficiency in your childhood.

Children suffering from a vitamin A deficiency are going to suffer from night blindness. This means that they cannot see clearly, or possibly not at all, when the light is dim.

A vitamin A deficiency is also capable of causing blindness in children, especially when they are young.

Adults are usually spread the extreme manifestations of these deficiency diseases. However, they are going to show symptoms like tiredness, reduced work capacity and poor concentration power. These are the direct results of iron deficiency.

A poor performance at both work and at home can possibly aggravate your irritation quotient and make both you and your family members, miserable.

Vitamin A deficiency also can manifest itself as night blindness. A teenager may not suffer from permanent eye damage, due to vitamin A deficiency, however, night blindness will definitely affect her movements at dawn and at dusk.

In adults, iodine deficiency can cause you to suffer from the enlargement of the thyroid. This is called a goiter.

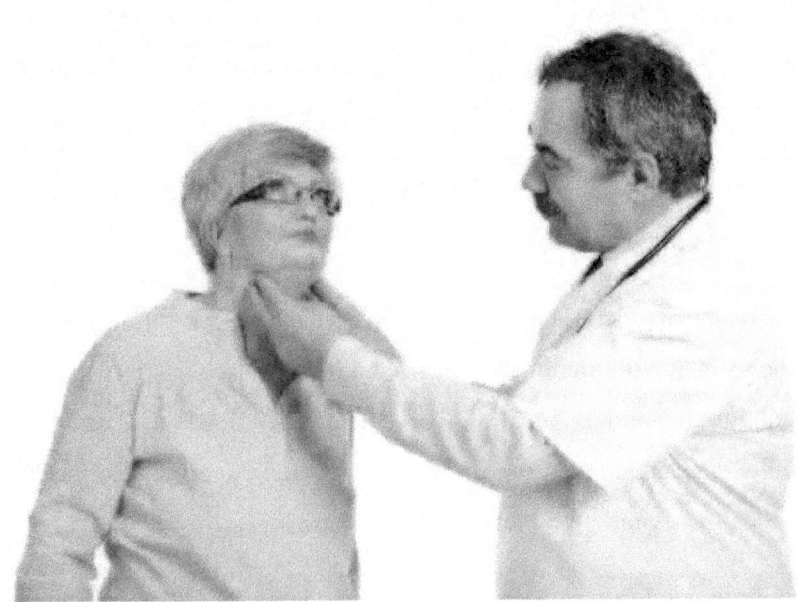

People living in the mountains normally suffer from iodine deficiency. I do, because I spent my childhood, far away from the sea, and from seafood rich in iodine. I do not suffer from a goiter, because one of the well-known salt packaging brands has been told by the government to add iodine to the salt before packing.

However, let me tell you this medieval story about how a king of a small state in the heels managed to use this iodine deficiency to good use.

In the 16th century, his land was overrun by invaders, and they decided to settle there. They made their palaces and their gardens with architects and planners brought over from their land. When they were already to bring in their courts, and their families, and their people, the king of that particular region got a really good idea.

He waited till all the aristocratic and dainty ladies of the court were settled in those beautiful palaces and gardens. And then he sent his native mountain people to work in the gardens and in the palaces as servants.

Each one of them was chosen specially by the King himself. And each one had an enlarged goiter.

Naturally, the aristocratic ladies were horrified. What was this, all the men and the women working in the gardens and in the palace had throats which were definitely not thin and swan like? Their eyes bulged out. They had difficulty in speaking, because the swelling around their throats affected their vocal cords and pronunciation.

The hill folk modestly said that there was something in the water, which affected them so. It was possible that the outsiders had some magic which would prevent them from suffering from this power in the water.

The "outsiders" were not having any! The ladies went first, gathering their children unto them, and disappearing in the night, back to their native land. The men stuck on for a couple of months, but wherever they looked, they saw people with an enlarged swelling around their throats.

And so they left too. They never came back to those conquered lands again. There was something there in the water!

And the king got the conquerors to build palaces and gardens in his land, and these beautiful gardens still exist today. So this is where intelligence rules over ignorance! A micronutrient deficiency is going to make you more prone to infections.

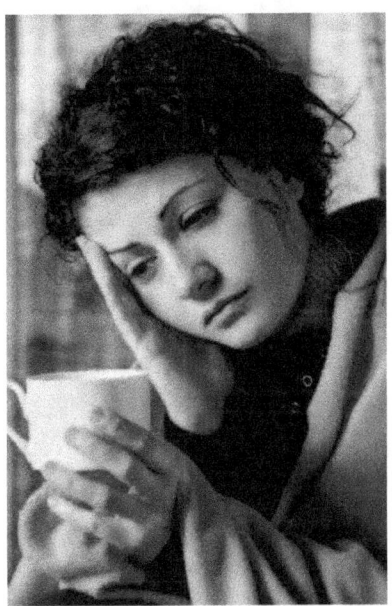

A micronutrient deficiency is going to affect your immunity system and make you more prone to cough, colds, and infections.

The worrying fact is that many of us do not know all about these deficiencies until the symptoms begin to affect our body systems. The symptoms may not appear visibly and that is why we do not bother much about any possible effect on our health. This also means that harm is being done to our bodies, even before we begin to get aware that our diet is inadequate.

Choosing the Best Diet

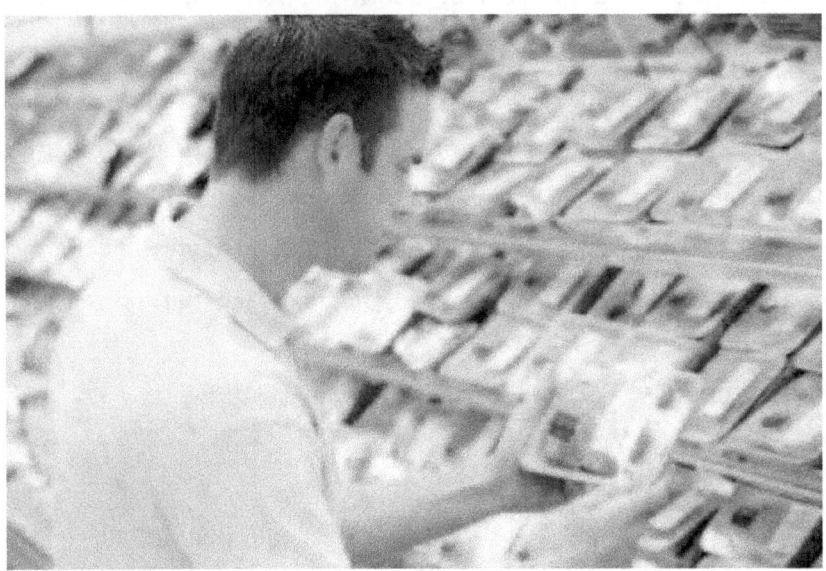

Many of us have this bad habit of sticking to just one food group, because we are so used to eating that particular food since childhood. Many of us do not eat greens because our parents never taught us that greens are important in keeping us healthy.

Or it is possible that they told us to eat carrots and eat our greens, because they were healthy for us. Which child likes to be told that he needs to eat something just because it is healthy for him? If our parents had said, do not eat these greens, because then you are going to look like the Green Giant, we would immediately have chomped down upon them.

So being a parent means you need inverse psychology. But sadly enough, a large majority of people, even those who considered themselves to be in the higher income bracket group and can eat lots of "healthy" food regularly, also suffer from vitamin A, iodine, and iron deficiency.

Every fifth person in the USA alone is suffering from a micronutrient deficiency. You say, how can that be, because people normally eat a very healthy diet rich in fruit, vegetables, and other healthy food groups, very often here. The thing is that many of these are processed or are grown with hormone enhancers. So they may have these vitamins, but in lesser quantities. Instead, your body is going to be subjected to growth hormones, which were injected by the gardeners to add bulk to the fruit and vegetables.

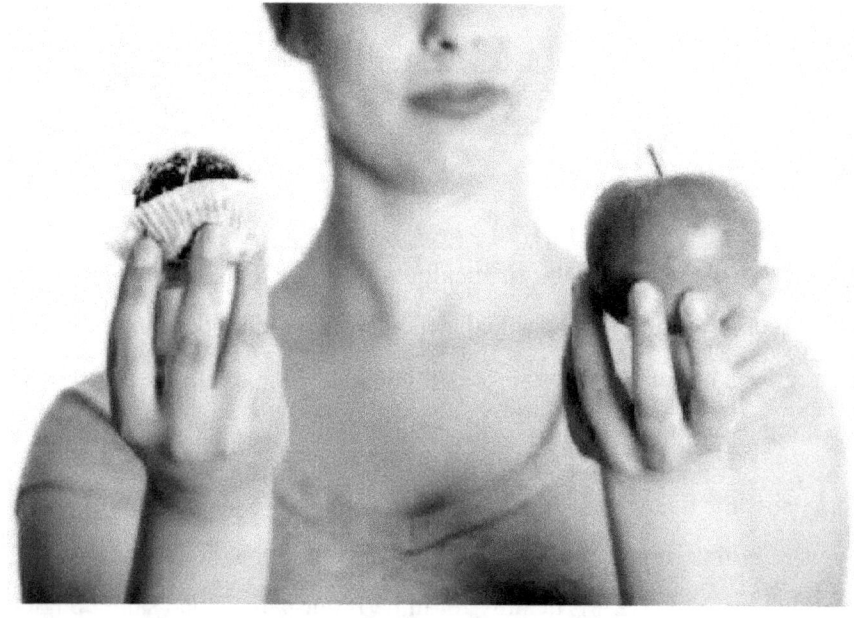

Apart from the nutritional value, your diet today is going to make all the difference between future health and possible sickness in the long run.

Every third, teenage girl, and every second child below six years is anemic due to iron deficiency. This is what researchers have found out. If a girl suffers from anemia in childhood, it is possible that she will not be able to bear children later in life.

It is estimated that more than 126 million people all over the world show some sort of iodine deficiency. Further, with every passing hour, another 10 children are born, being physically and mentally "retarded" due to iodine deficiency.

At least 4 – 8% of children in the USA suffer from some sort of disorder due to deficiency of vitamin A. You are going to be surprised to hear that, because you say that you are feeding your children healthy and nutritious food, so how could they suffer from a vitamin A deficiency?

Is it possible that you are feeding your children with branded supplements and energy drinks, which supposedly give your children the necessary nutrients needed to keep them healthy? Believe it or not, I noticed many of my friends in the West with these branded drinks on their breakfast table. They also had breakfast cereals "enhanced with vitamins and minerals".

I can say very stridently, that all of this is a marketing stunt. The moment you hear a superstar or a celebrity endorsing something which has been enhanced with minerals, you need to ask yourself, what did they take out that they needed to add something else to compensate?

So you may want to know whether fortified foods are really beneficial or not?

Fortified Foods

The jury is out on that one. Being an advocate of natural foods, it is possible that I am prejudiced against fortified foods. But many times, dietitians want you to complement healthy eating habits with fortified foods such as flour with added iron, cooking oils with vitamin A, salt with iodine, etc. this is a simple and effective way of ensuring an adequate intake of these micronutrients.

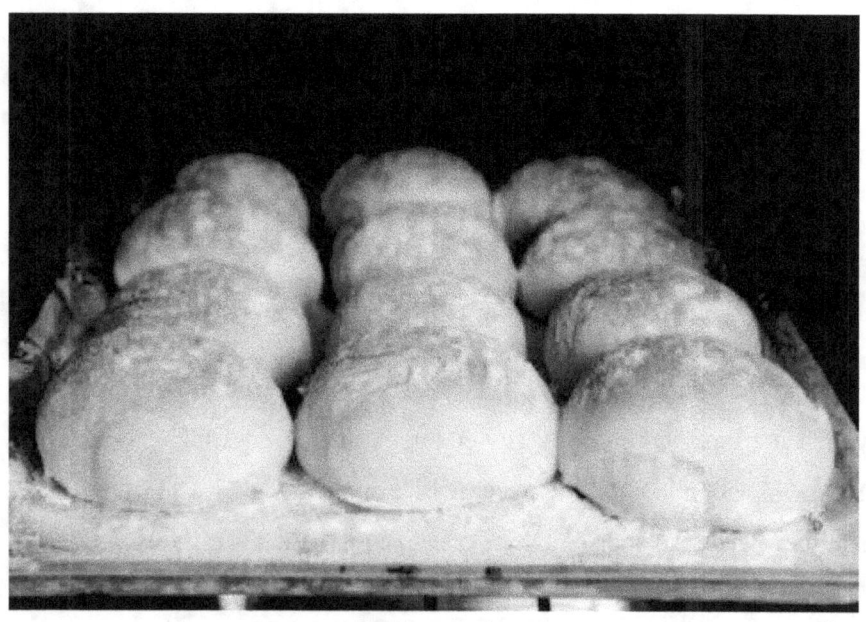

Many bakers use fortified flour in baking, nowadays.

Remember that these are not expensive brand names. They are not enhanced food items or breakfast cereals. They are food items you eat every day in your daily diet.

Consumption of fortified foods does not require any change in your food habits. They are particularly relevant in situations when you want convenience foods that reduce your drudgery and at the same time provide proper nutrition.

In the early 1900s, salt was iodized in Switzerland. During the 1930s and 1940s, milk was fortified with vitamin A and flour with Iron in Europe and North America. Over the last 40 years, several other nutritional definitions have been eliminated in this way.

Today fortified foods provide at least 30% of the daily requirements of vitamin A in Western diets.

Preventing Micronutrient Deficiency

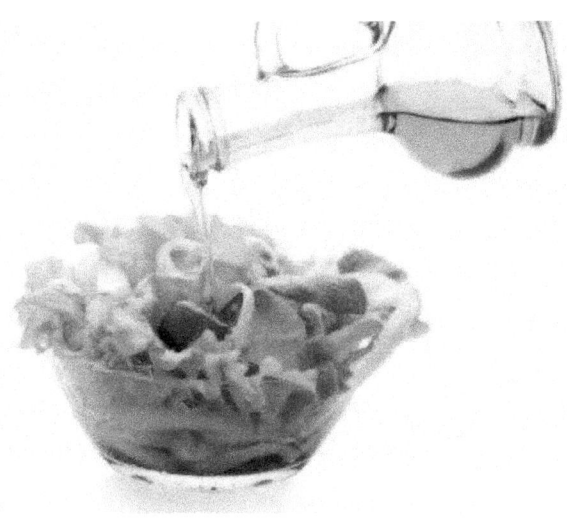

Well, the answer is a very practical one. All you have to do is consume a balanced diet containing adequate amounts of micronutrient rich foods. This is easily going to prevent any sort of micronutrient deficiency.

A number of foods are rich in iron and vitamin A. I will be giving you a food table where you can find all the foods which are going to help prevent hidden hunger. Apart from seafood, there are very few other foods which are good sources of iodine.

That is why you have to make sure that your family eats lots of vegetables, particularly, Greenleaf, you vegetables which are rich in iron and vitamin A at both lunch and dinner.

Make sure that all the members of your family, children, you and the elders combine this diet with lots of milk/milk products and if you are non–vegetarian, have eggs, chicken, meat and fish frequently.

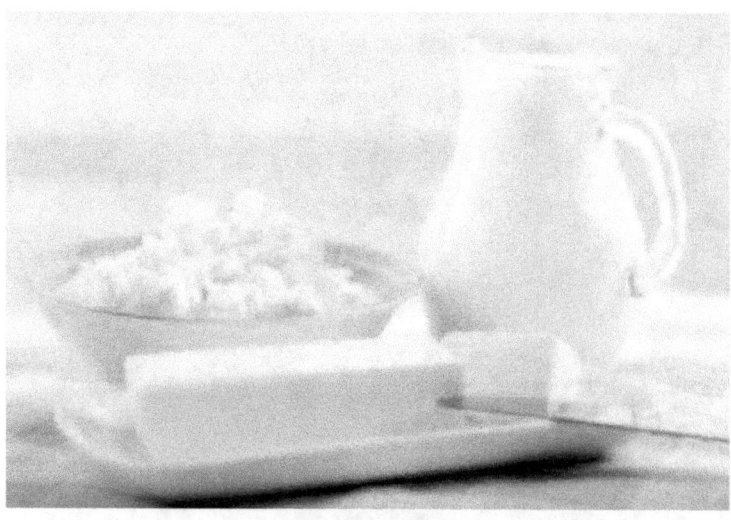

I found a very disturbing trend being followed in the West where a campaign against dairy products and milk products is being propagated as something which is not necessary for adults. I was surprised to hear that, especially when somebody said that dairy products like butter and cheese and butter milk would not be drunk by a number of adults because of health reasons and for weight reasons.

Use some common sense. What would you rather be, a little plump and healthy or totally obsessed with your weight, and growing unhealthy. Just because you are not eating healthy food, including milk, butter, cheese, cottage cheese and butter milk, just because some skeletal and skinny person advocates that?

Foods rich in vitamin A and iron –

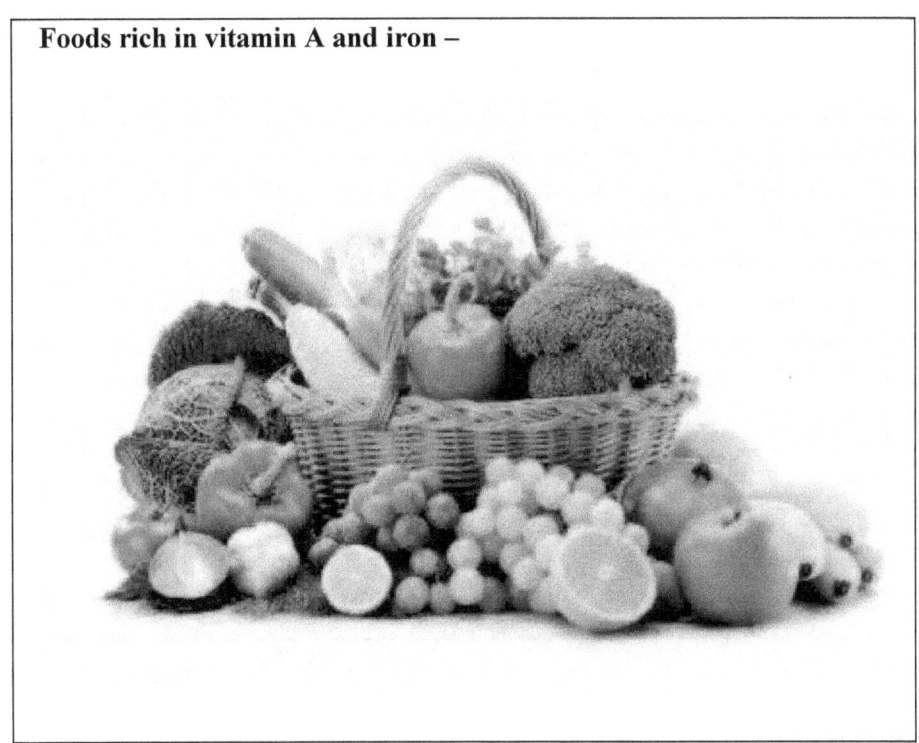

Both vegetables and animal foods are good sources of iron and vitamin A.	Vitamin A	Iron
Green leafy vegetables – parsley, coriander, fenugreek, cabbage, spinach, mint, radish leaves, mustard	Yes	Yes
Orange/yellow fruit, like Papayas and mangoes.	Yes	–
Yellow/orange vegetables – pumpkins, carrots, etc.	Yes	–
Milk and milk products – butter, butter, milk, yogurt, cottage cheese	Yes	–
Eggs	Yes	–
Meat , especially liver	Yes	Yes
Cereals and their flours, especially wheat, barley, etc.	–	Yes
Pulses and beans especially sprouted beans	–	Yes
Dates, molasses	–	Yes

Conclusion

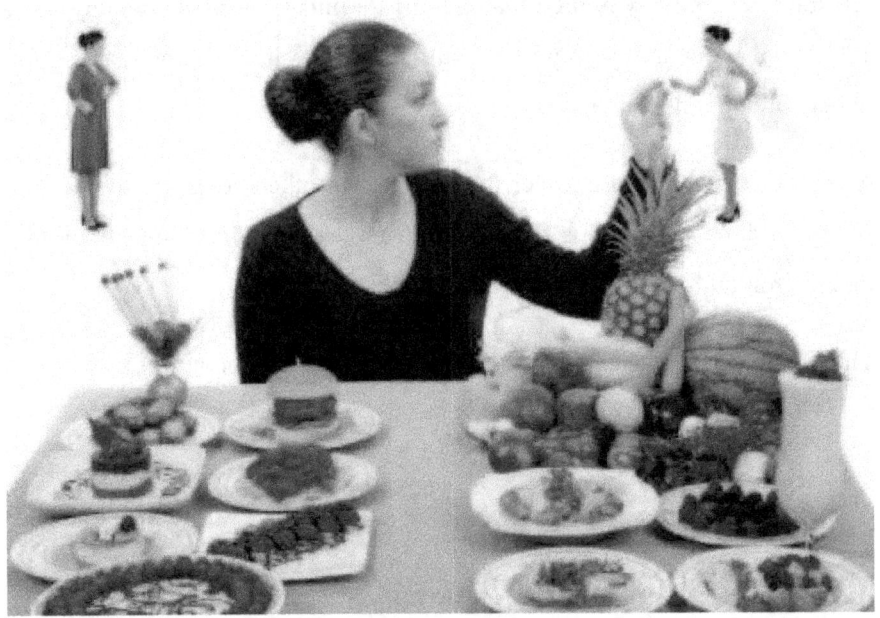

Bad eating habits can cause a micronutrient deficiency. However, you may suppose that you are eating sensibly and still suffer from this deficiency, if you do not eat the proper foods in proper quantities at every meal.

This book has given you plenty of information about how you can prevent any sort of micronutrient deficiency in your family and in you. Suffering from hidden hunger can easily be prevented if you know all about it, and you can take steps that that does not occur in your vicinity.

Remember that a number of us keep eating indiscriminately and in large quantities, just because the food is there. That is the reason why we suffer from problems related to a huge food intake. However, when we eat sensibly we can be reassured that even if the intake is comparatively large, at least we are eating the right food stuffs, at the right time, and that is going to benefit us in the long run.

A number of countries all over the world have taken steps to provide their people with food, which is fortified with minerals, and vitamins, including iodine, iron and vitamin A.

These include salt, wheat flour, and their products, and breakfast cereals.

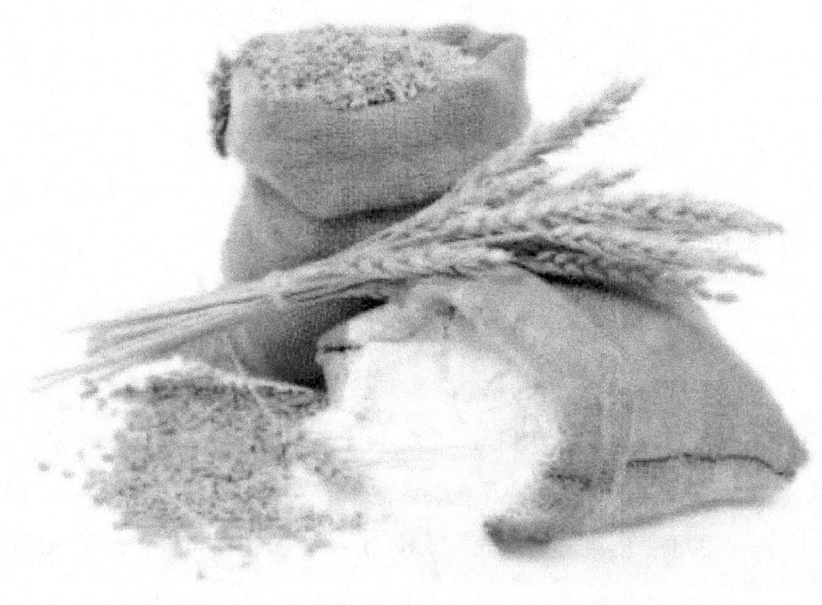

There is a major category of breakfast cereals, which are being sold after being fortified with micronutrients. Naturally, as breakfast is a very important meal of the day, it is going to contribute considerably to our daily nutrient intake. Some of the cereals also have calcium and zinc in them.

Cooking oils – in some countries all over the world, cooking oils are fortified with vitamins A and D. This trend started in the 1950s. Margarine was fortified with vitamin A during the Second World War and that is still being followed, till date.

Milk and Jam products are also being fortified with vitamins in many parts of the world today.

That is because in many countries the government as well as food industry has realized that food fortification is going to benefit people from all the economic strata and keep them healthy.

Also, in many countries, research is being conducted to check the feasibility of fortifying salt with iron along with iodine as well as milk, sugar, and Tea with vitamin A. That is because these items are consumed by almost any consumer of which you can think.

Fortified rice has also come in the market in many parts of the world today. But I find this ironic because this rice is processed first. And in this procedure, all the essential nutrients, which are present, naturally in the rice before the processing was done, get removed. So first we remove the natural nutrients by processing the rice and then we add fortifying agents in order to supplement those natural nutrients!

What fools these mortals be.

These fortified foods are meant for the general public. So whenever you go shopping for food, remember to check the label and see what you are eating. Does the food give you a proper an additional micronutrient, if you are eating packaged food and processed food.

If the answer is yes, which are additional micronutrient has been added? Is it an essential micronutrient like vitamin A, iron and iodine or is it just a gimmick to gain sales?

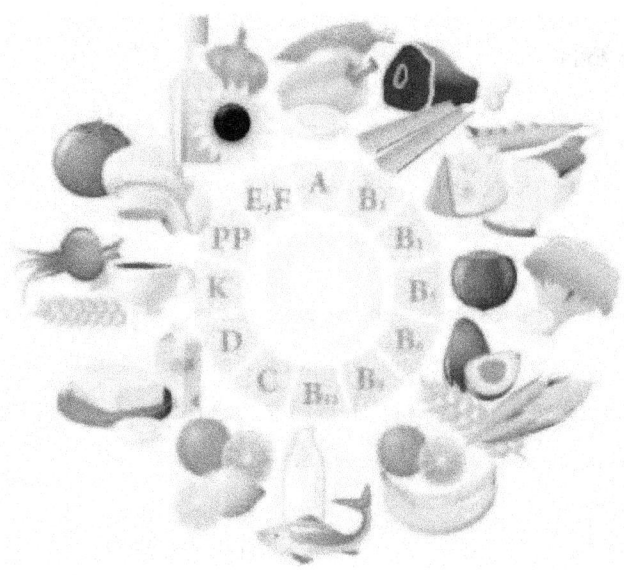

Only when you are completely aware and informed, can you make the correct choices in your shopping and thus ensure the continuous good health of your family.

Live Long and Prosper!

Author Bio

Dueep Jyot Singh is a Management and IT Professional who managed to gather Postgraduate qualifications in Management and English and Degrees in Science, French and Education while pursuing different enjoyable career options like being an hospital administrator, IT,SEO and HRD Database Manager/ trainer, movie , radio and TV scriptwriter, theatre artiste and public speaker, lecturer in French, Marketing and Advertising, ex-Editor of Hearts On Fire (now known as Solstice) Books Missouri USA, advice columnist and cartoonist, publisher and Aviation School trainer, ex-moderator on Medico.in, banker, student councilor ,travelogue writer … among other things!

One fine morning, she decided that she had enough of killing herself by Degrees and went back to her first love -- writing. It's more enjoyable! She already has 48 published academic and 14 fiction- in- different- genre books under her belt.

When she is not designing websites or making Graphic design illustrations for clients , she is browsing through old bookshops hunting for treasures, of which she has an enviable collection – including R.L. Stevenson, O.Henry, Dornford Yates, Maurice Walsh, De Maupassant, Victor Hugo, Sapper, C.N. Williamson, "Bartimeus" and the crown of her collection- Dickens "The Old Curiosity Shop," and "Martin Chuzzlewit" and so on… Just call her "Renaissance Woman") - collecting herbal remedies, acting like Universal Helping Hand/Agony Aunt, or escaping to her dear mountains for a bit of exploring, collecting herbs and plants and trekking.

Check out some of the other JD-Biz Publishing books

Gardening Series on Amazon

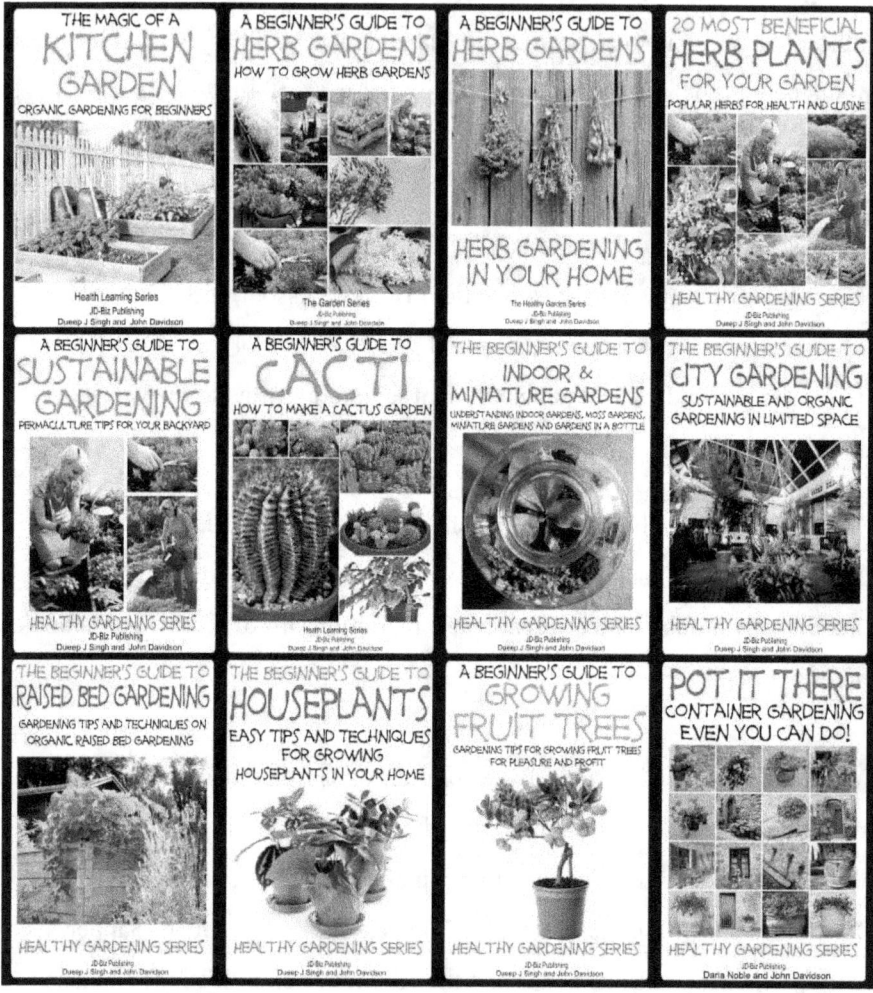

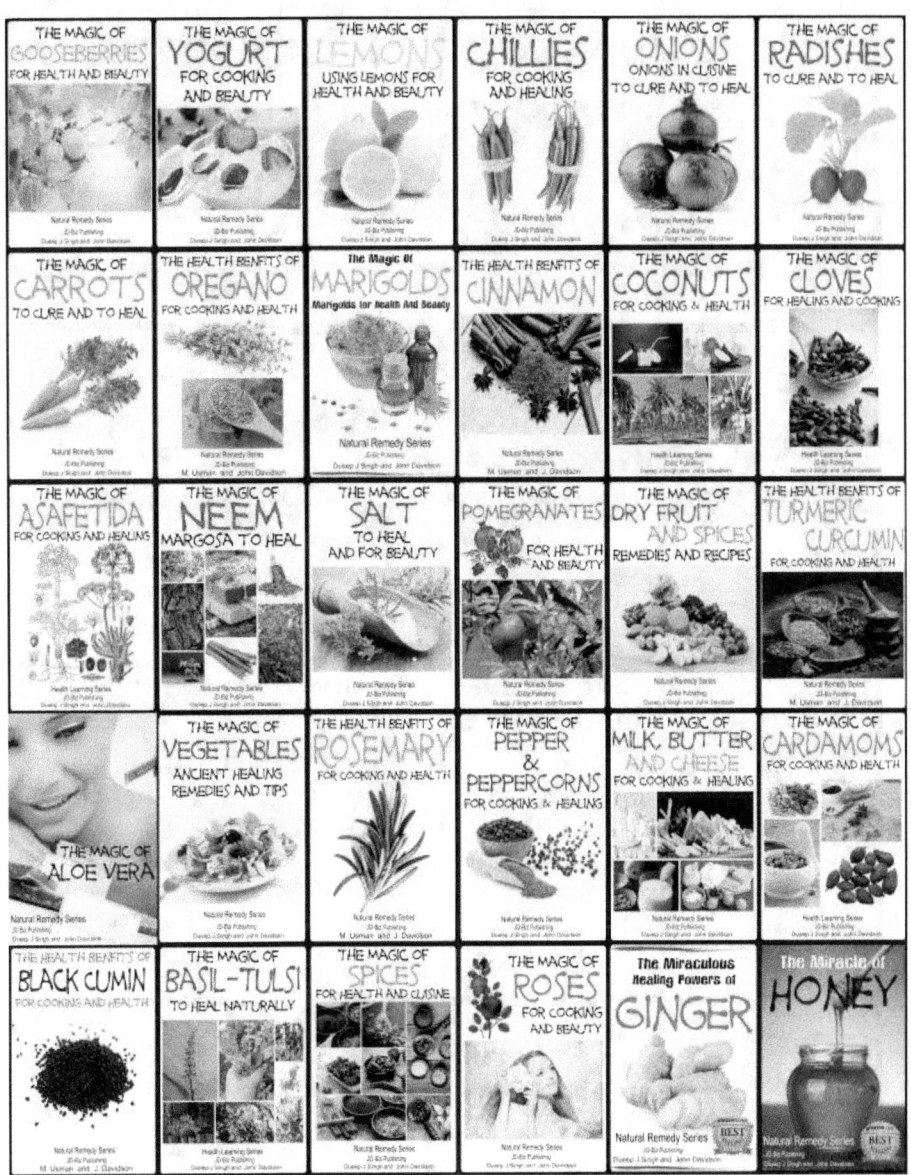

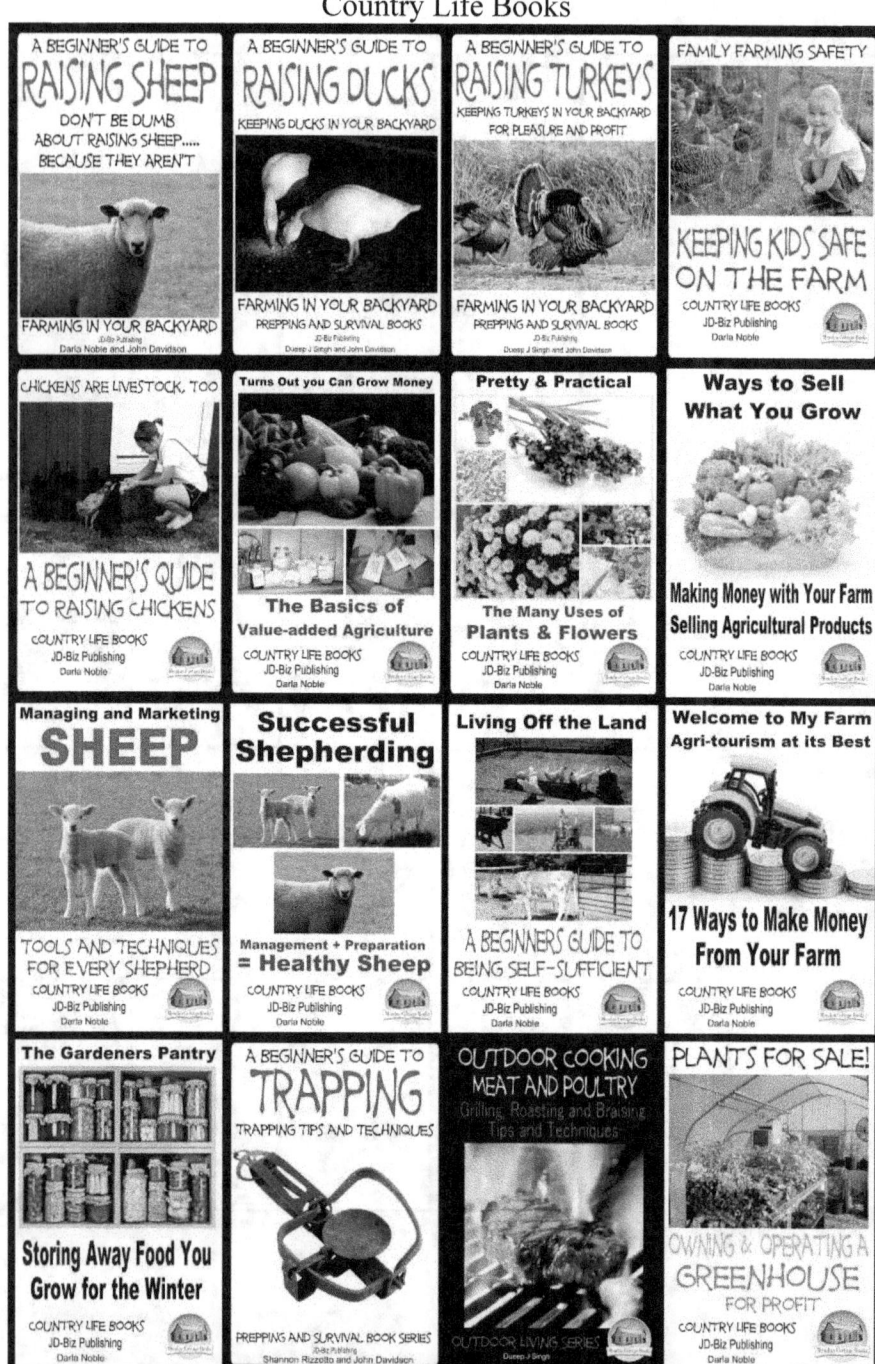

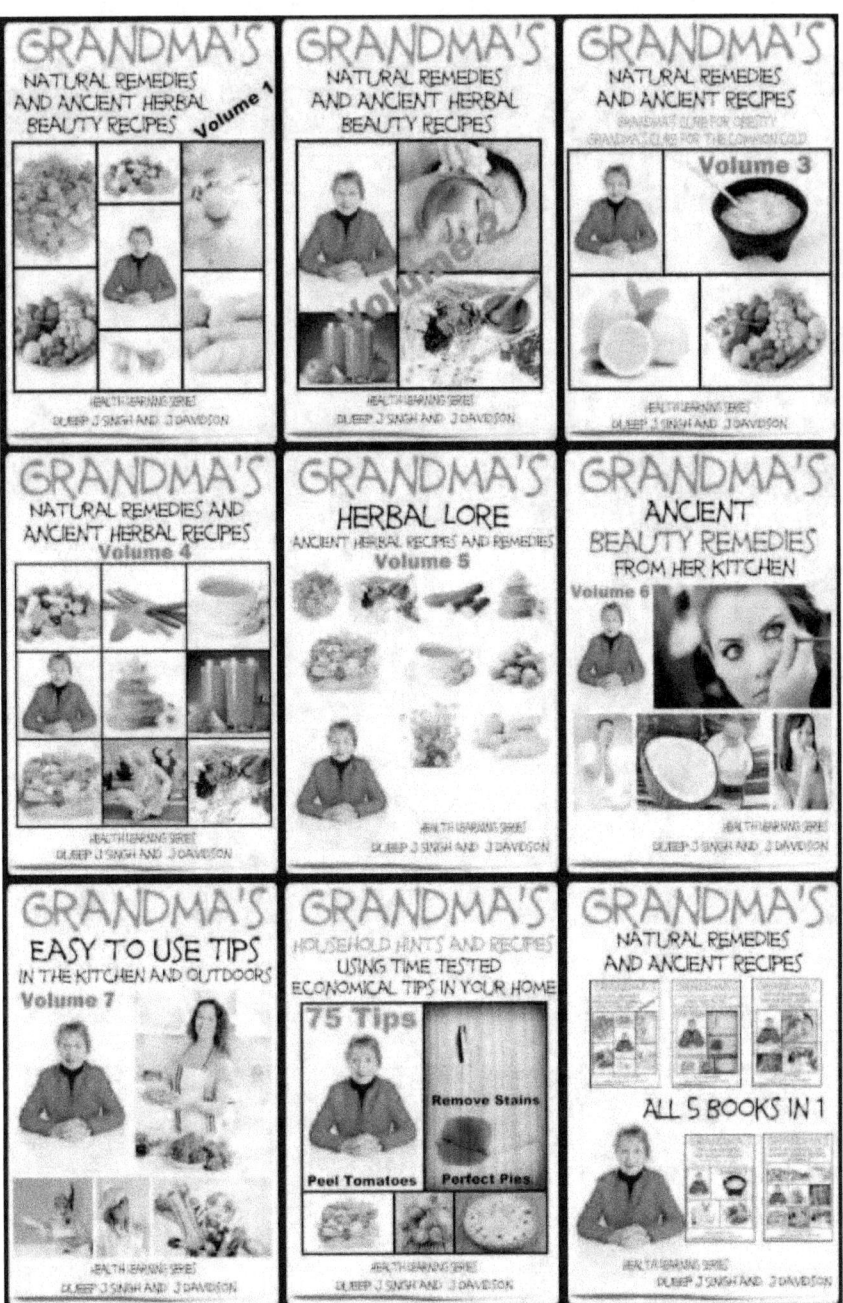

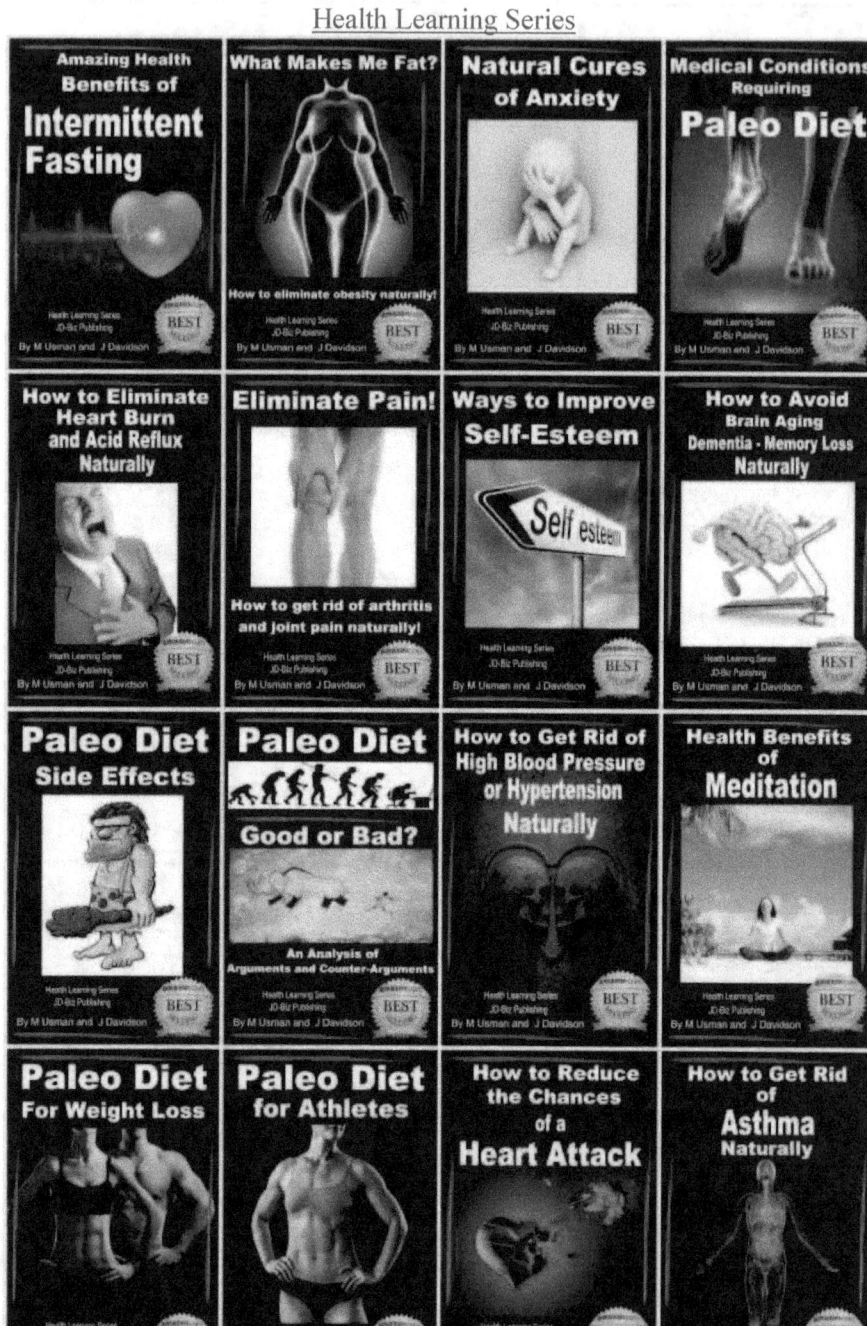

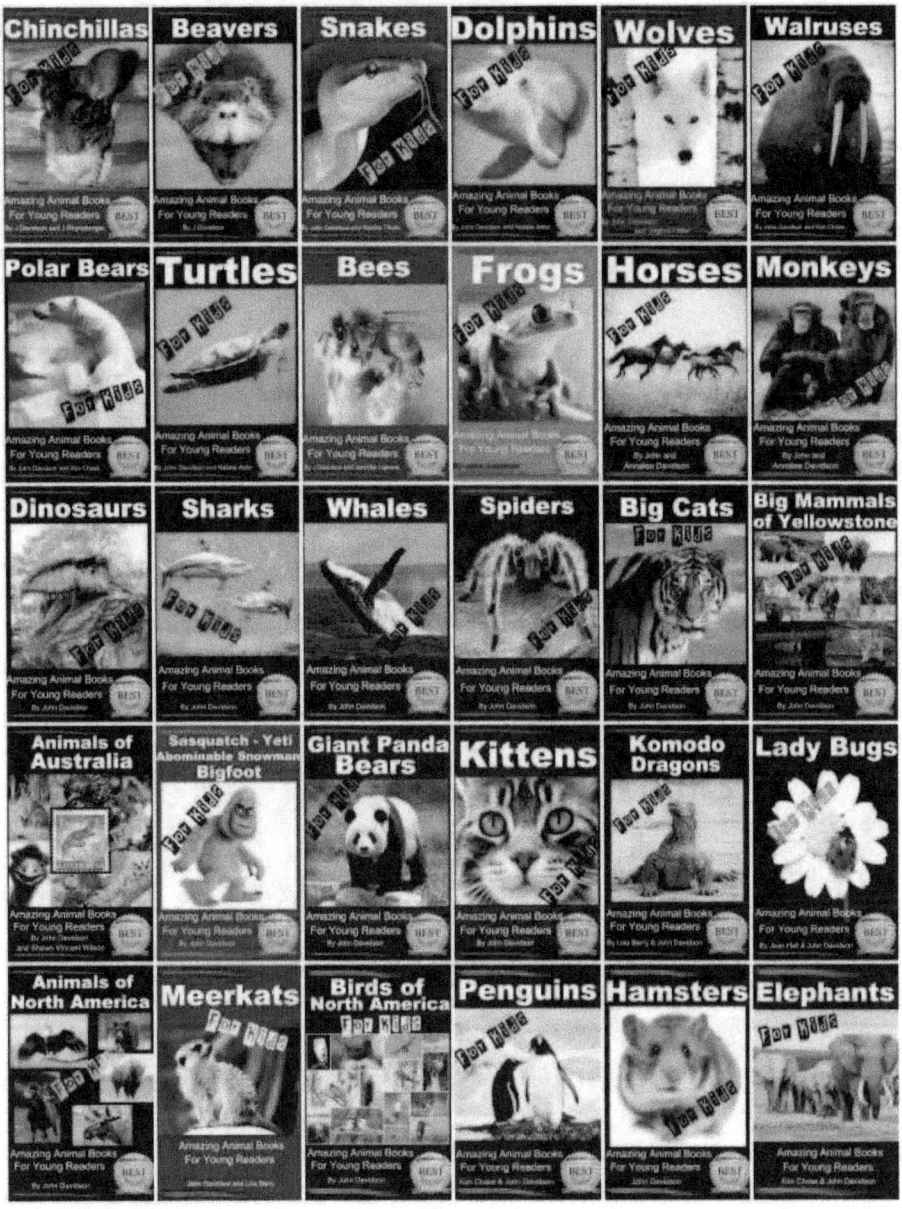

Learn To Draw Series

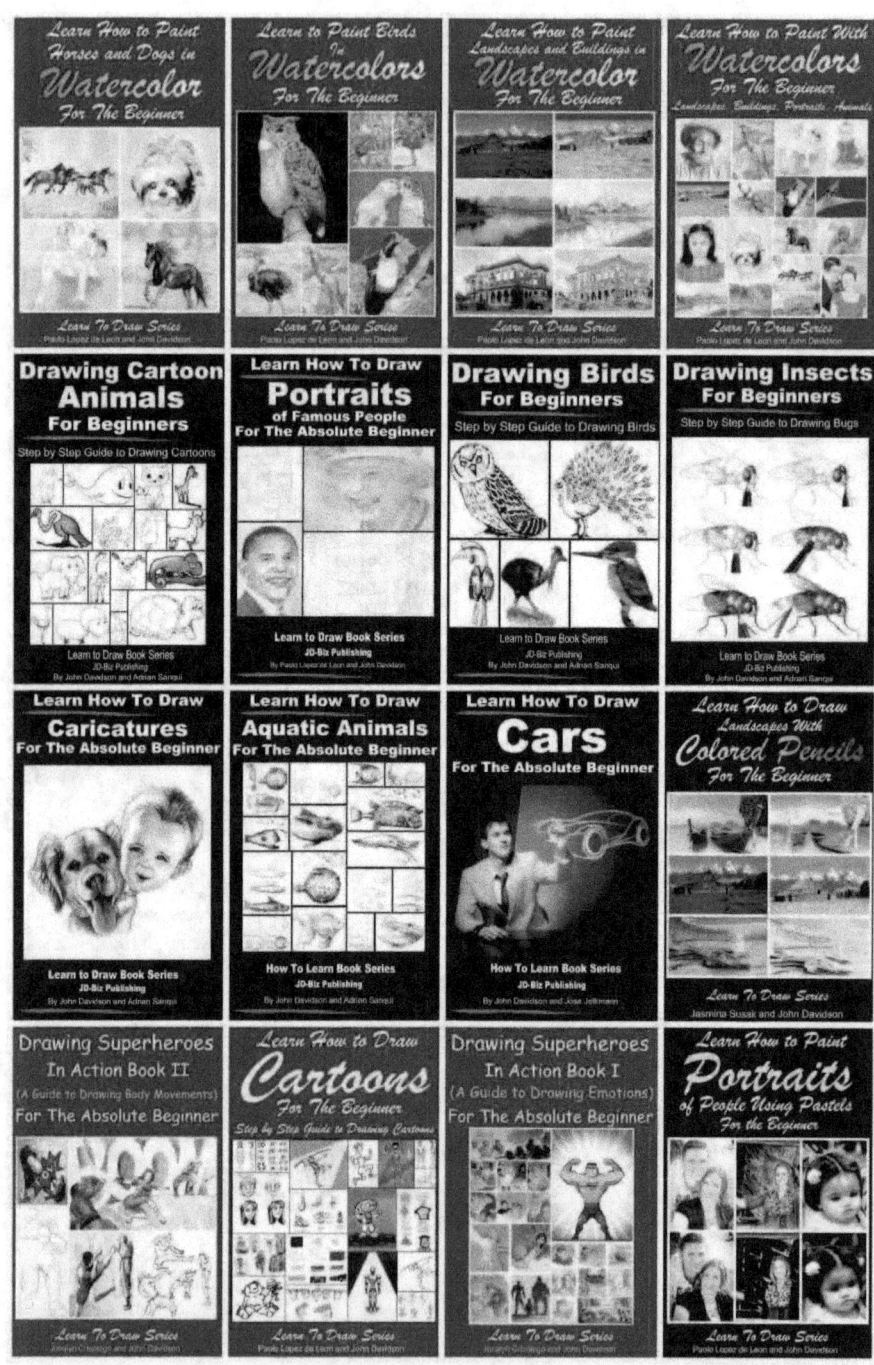

How to Build and Plan Books

Entrepreneur Book Series

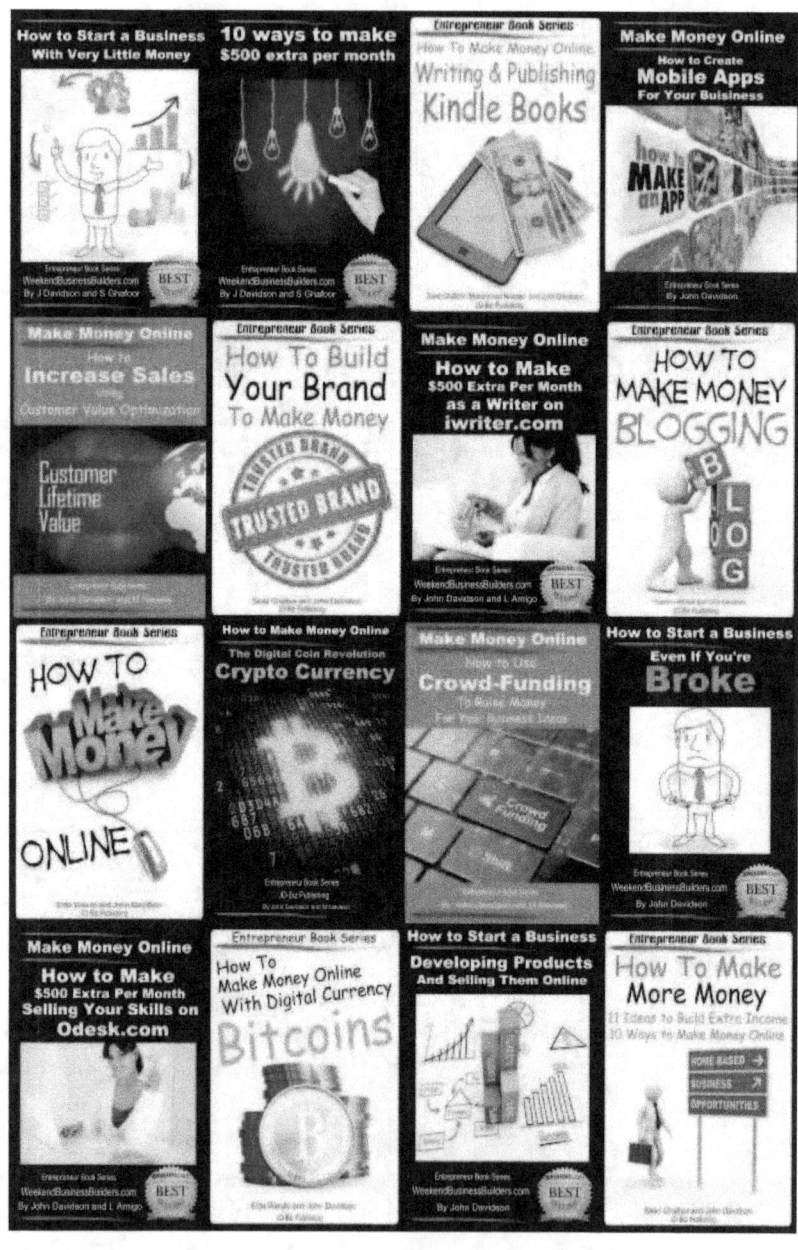

Our books are available at

1. Amazon.com

2. Barnes and Noble

3. Itunes

4. Kobo

5. Smashwords

6. Google Play Books

Publisher

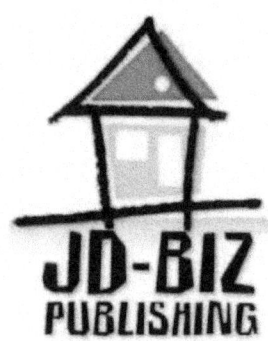

JD-Biz Corp

P O Box 374

Mendon, Utah 84325

http://www.jd-biz.com/

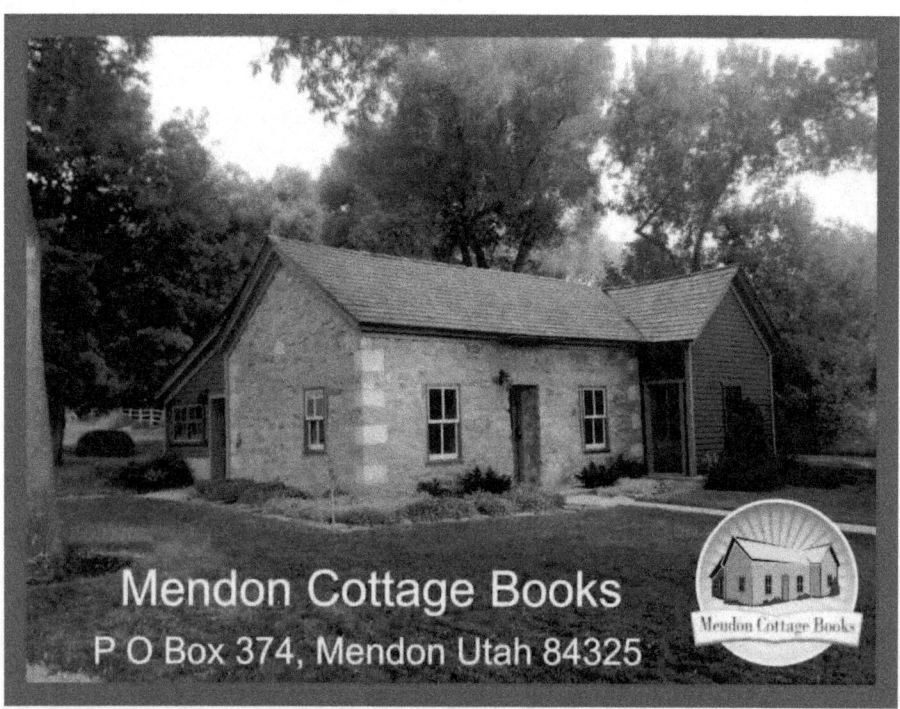

Mendon Cottage Books

P O Box 374, Mendon Utah 84325